I0712043

MEMORY FAIL

LINDA LOPRASERT

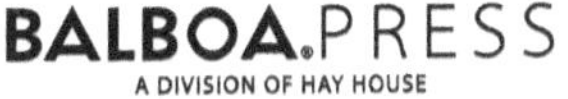

BALBOA.PRESS
A DIVISION OF HAY HOUSE

Balboa Press books may be ordered through booksellers or by contacting:

Balboa Press
A Division of Hay House
1663 Liberty Drive
Bloomington, IN 47403
www.balboapress.com.au
AU TFN: 1 800 844 925 (Toll Free inside Australia)
AU Local: (02) 8310 7086 (+61 2 8310 7086 from outside Australia)

Print information available on the last page.

ISBN: 979-8-7652-0016-2 (sc)
ISBN: 979-8-7652-0015-5 (e)

Library of Congress Control Number: 2024915442

Balboa Press rev. date: 08/01/2024

Contents

Preface

Throughout this book, I take you through my cancer journey, from diagnosis through to treatment, and post treatment. I lay it out bare for you, by reading this book from beginning to end you will experience what it's like to have brain cancer, and some of the weird and wacky experiences, or "memory fails" as I like to call it that became part of life. A note however I'd like to make is that this is *my brain cancer journey*. Every cancer, every patient has their own individual experience. I know this as I have met many other brain cancer patients who have had brain cancer, or brain trauma, and each and every individual I have met experience different symptoms and issues. Everyone is unique, everybody is different.

The purpose of this book is to share my journey and I hope that it will reach someone/ anyone that is experiencing something similar, and to know that *you are not alone*. If I had picked up this book whilst I was lying in my hospital bed, I would have felt hope, felt that there was a positive end to it all. So, I encourage you to please share this book with anyone who may be going through something difficult, and would benefit in seeing the light at the end of the tunnel.

Chapter 1: Life "Pre-cancer"

Life pre-cancer was amazing. It really was. I had it all.

I graduated university with a first class honours in finance. I had a well paying job; I was making 6 figures in my early 20's, I was pretty proud of myself. I was in a stable, long-term relationship. I was living in the city, within walking distance of my workplace, bars, restaurants, shops… I had it all, I really did.

I enjoyed life. Friday nights and Saturday nights, you would find me at one of the nightclubs, bars, or restaurants around the Sydney CBD. On public holidays, I'd be away; on a weekend trip around NSW, on a domestic trip around Australia, or an international holiday.

I did all of this with my friends, of which I had plenty of at the time.

Every weekend was choc-a-block busy with drinking, partying, brunching, exploring… with friends. My early 20's, my "pre cancer" days were so much fun.

That's one thing I am thankful for, that I was able to live my life, go out and party and do stupid things… all before I was hit with the C-bomb at the age of 26. Because, from that point onwards, my entire life changed. *My entire life.*

Chapter 2: Something's wrong

There were many signs, many instances that indicated to me, that made me know deep down, without a doubt, that something was very *very* wrong. I chose to ignore these signs for as long as I could, until I got to a point where I could not ignore them anymore, I knew I *had* to see a Doctor.

The first sign that something was wrong was my memory. At the time, I was working as a client services executive and one of the key reasons I was doing so well in my job was my memory; I would be able to recall immediately which client was buying what product and for how much and who the key contact was at that company. I'd be able to multi-task between tasks with no effort at all. I was always on the ball. I was a star employee.

Then one day, I just started dropping the ball on everything. I would 'forget' to do tasks that were assigned to me. I would repeat the same questions. I was not me. I could feel it. My manager could feel it.

Aside from the obvious memory issue, I also had a few hallucinations. There's one I remember very clearly, even to this day, and even to this day it brings goosebumps to my arms. I have a memory of walking down the street, chatting with someone. Then I turn around, and the street was empty. It was a scary feeling, and it was at that point, the hallucinations along with the horrible memory that I finally accepted that something was seriously wrong. So, I booked an appointment with my Doctor. Upon hearing my symptoms, my Doctor immediately sent me for an MRI of the brain.

A MRI is very serious. It's not a routine test that a GP sends their patients to. It was serious, and I knew it.

I don't remember the scan.
I remember the result.
I remember seeing the result.
The Doctor put the scan up on one of those translucent screens in order to see the MRI film, which is similar to an X-ray film.
He pointed to a large grey mass, a round shape, about the size of a golf ball, in my brain.
That was my brain tumour.

I think I went blank.
I went numb.
Brain tumour? Me? Really?

Chapter 3: Biopsy

The next step was to get a biopsy done, for the Doctors to understand what they were dealing with.

In order for the biopsy to be done, part of my hair was shaven off, to allow the surgeon to make an incision point.

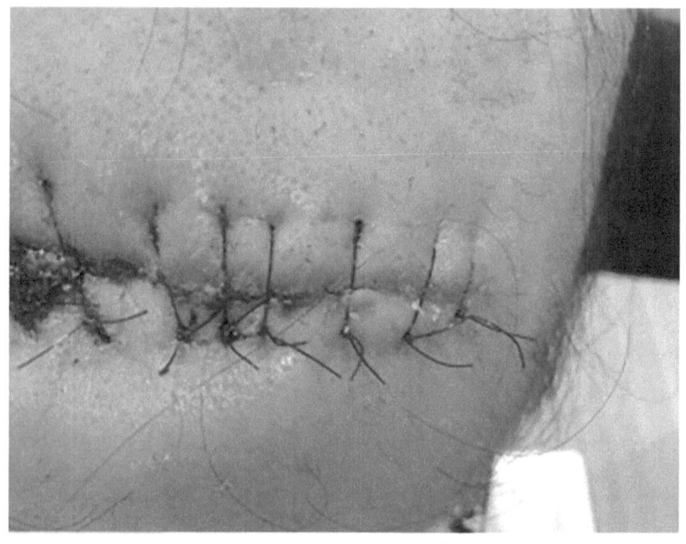

Incision point, stitched up post biopsy

The biopsy went well, a sample was taken for the Doctors to take to the laboratory for investigation and testing.

Meanwhile, my hair started growing back around the incision point.

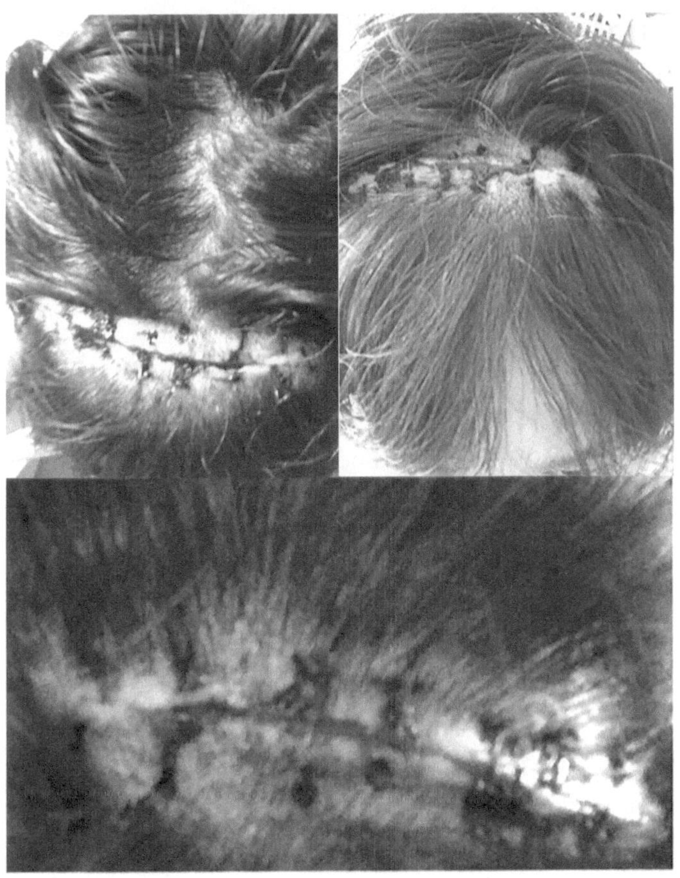

Incision point, hair growing back

I was instructed to *not* get the incision point, and anywhere around the incision point wet. If I were to take a shower, I was to wear a shower cap, a very secure one, wrapped up.

I followed orders, and when showering, wore a shower

cap. However, there was still a little moisture that crept through. That was bad.

The feeling I had was similar to a kettle boiling, but on my head. Yes, that sounds very strange to say, but that's what it felt like.

Needless to say, I had an infection, from water getting onto my wound.

Lesson learnt.

No more showers until my head wound/ incision point was 100% healed. There was no way I was going to risk another hospital stay. I would rather be shower-less and smelly for a few days, than risk another infection.

So, no showers it was.

Chapter 4: Diagnosis

Germinoma of the third ventricle.

That is what the biopsy revealed that I had.

Germinoma of the third ventricle. Germinoma. Germinoma. Germinoma. That's all that was going through my head. I remember thinking, it has a name now, it's real. *It's real,*

The first thing I did when I got home was jump on the internet to research this, what was this, what was this *Germinoma of the third ventricle.*

Of course, Google didn't help. It just made it worse, spitting out hundreds of webpages talking about things I knew nothing about. It was information overload. Instead of making me feel more informed and better, it made me feel *worse.*

I just wanted to know what was in my brain, how it got there, how long it had been there for, how to get rid of it, how to get my life back…. Ok… there were *lots* of things I wanted to know. Questions were running through my head.

Chapter 5: Treatment and being 'homeless'

I was told that I was *lucky*, because the tumour I had, a germinoma of the third ventricle, is highly sensitive to treatment and the success and survival rate is very high.

Oh great, I thought. I got brain cancer, but at least I was lucky enough to get a highly treatable form of brain cancer.

My treatment plan was given to me:

- 3 rounds of chemotherapy, each round to be 1 week long. I was to stay in the hospital for each of those rounds.
- Following my 3 rounds of chemotherapy, I would then be given radiation therapy. The radiation would be directed to my brain, to be administered every day for 10 minutes, for 1 month.

All of this happened over the space of one-and-a-half years.

Whilst doing my cancer treatment, I was also being shuffled between homes. To provide some context, when I was diagnosed with cancer, I was renting an apartment in the city, sharing with a friend. Obviously, after my cancer diagnosis, I had to give up that apartment as I no longer had the income to pay rent, and I needed daily care.

I ended up being shipped between my Mum's place and my brother's place. It was difficult, I didn't have my own room, my things were split between 2 places, I didn't feel like I had a permanent home.

At the time, I felt resentful about this, I felt that if I had a loving, caring family home to recover in, that would have helped to speed up my recovery.

All of my personal belongings, from the apartment I was renting in the city, had been packed up for me whilst I was in hospital. I presume it was my Mum that did this for me, to this day I have not asked her. I try not to talk or think too much about my treatment days.

It was around this time that I was being very tough on myself, and feeling that everything was *against* me instead of *for* me. It was at this point in time that I first started having suicidal thoughts. My brain was thinking, I don't have any friends, I don't have a partner, I'm a burden on my family, my memory is horrible, and I have no prospects of finding a boyfriend (or husband!), or even a job for that matter. What was the point of it all? I might as well end *my* suffering and let everyone else, meaning my family, off the hook, they can stop worrying and caring for me, and just live their lives. These were the horrid thoughts going through my brain. And, what was even more horrid, was I actually started to put a list together of the most *painless* and *effective* ways to die. I wanted it to be painless, because I am scared of pain, and I wanted it to be effective, because life would be even worse if my suicide attempt was unsuccessful, I'd *definitely* end up in the mental ward. I thought about it really hard, and in my mind, the best way to die would be for someone to shoot me. Point blank, shoot me. *I needed to find a hitman, a hitman on myself.* Even writing that now sounds so scary, and something a lunatic would say. Well, that was me. It really was. I really went on my laptop and searched 'hitman' in Google, along with a few other phrases, about how to get one in Australia. To my disappointment, my research showed me that because guns are not legal in Australia, hiring a hitman is not something that's readily available in Australia. I'm glad that was the outcome of my absolutely ludicrous, crazy research. Yes, in hindsight, I can say that about my own actions; *hiring a hitman on myself?* It's so ludicrous, and absurd, and downright crazy that I'm not sure whether I should share so much detail in my book.

Chapter 5a: Chemotherapy, in detail

The thought of chemotherapy scared me. All I knew about chemotherapy was what I saw on sit-coms on TV. The patient would be attached to a machine, and when they're not attached to the machine they are vomiting and losing their hair.

And that's all I could picture for myself as well; vomiting and losing my hair. Not a nice picture.

Well, thanks to the advancements in science, vomiting was not an issue. Over the years, our very smart Doctors had developed an anti-nausea drug, so prior to each chemotherapy session, I would be given "the magic pill" as I'd like to call it, and viola, no nausea! In that sense, chemotherapy was pretty easy. For about 30 minutes (yes, only 30 minutes) of the day, I would be hooked up to the chemotherapy machine which would pump the drugs into me. During that time, I could do whatever I wanted, even walk around (the machine was on wheels, easily transportable).

Another thing about staying in hospital is all the injections you're given. I/ my arm did not respond well. I was black, blue and purple.

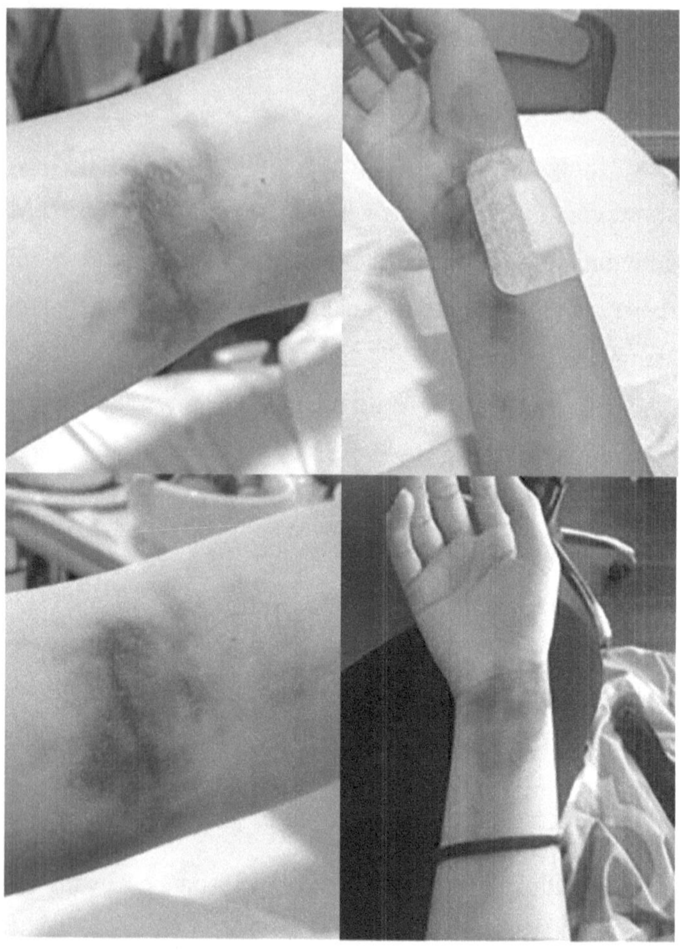

My black and blue arms as a result of daily injections

Losing your hair however, that was a real thing. It was a real thing that I was in denial about. I have always had long hair. I loved my long hair. I was asked whether I wanted to cut it short prior to chemotherapy starting, so that it wouldn't be so confronting when my hair would start to fall out; short hair = less hair to fall out, makes sense. But, I was in denial, I said I would be fine. Well, after my first round of chemotherapy, I understood what it was like for your hair to fall out. As I said, I had long hair, I loved it. I was in the shower washing my hair, running my fingers through my hair with shampoo. Oh dear... the amount of hair that came out, it was like a small animal died in the shower with me. I'm surprised the drain did not become permanently clogged.

Needless to say, I made an appointment with the hair dresser the very next day.

I stayed in the public hospital, sharing a room (and bathroom!) with 3 other people. It was not pleasant, but it's what has to be done under the public healthcare system. I kept myself occupied with reading and watching TV shows (I always brought my laptop with me to my chemotherapy sessions).

Hospital food, by no surprise, is very un-exciting and bland. I was lucky enough to always have home-cooked food brought to me by my family. I felt well cared for.

Chapter 5b: Radiation therapy, in detail

The final step of my treatment. Just one more month to go. To go to what, I found myself thinking sometimes. To go back to normal life? Go job searching, to 'friend' searching seeing as I'd lost most of my friends, to go back to living at home with my mum?

Stop it! I would tell myself. So many people get cancer, and so many people don't survive to tell the tale. I am beating this cancer. I should be happy, not worrying about insignificant things! That's what I told myself.

Radiation therapy itself was quite simple, and luckily for me, I didn't experience any side effects.

The procedure was, every day, for 30 days, I would need to go into Royal North Shore Hospital to get 10 minutes of radiation treatment, directed at where the tumour was sitting in my brain. This was done by strapping my head down, and lying still for 10 minutes. Pre work was done here, where they made a custom fit mold to fit my head, a mask in effect, which is what I was strapped into for each radiation session. Luckily, I didn't have any issues with claustrophobia, because it was a *very* tight fit, to ensure there was absolutely no movement, so that the radiation rays would target the correct areas. It made me think, I/ we all are so lucky to live in such a modernised world where medicine is so advanced.

Chapter 6: Why me

This chapter contains stories of parts of my cancer journey that I am *not* proud of, but it was a part of my journey nonetheless, so it needs to be shared to make the story complete.

I played the blame game. Why me. Why did I have to get cancer? What did I do wrong? I played the blame game. I was angry. I was angry at whoever, whatever gave me brain cancer. I was very angry. I was that angry person on the street swearing at everyone and anyone. I even lashed out at my nearest and dearest, my friends and family, the ones that were there to help me, to support me.

But I was too angry to care. I was angry beyond words. I was angry at the universe. And I didn't care who knew. I wanted everyone to know.

Well. All this did was push everyone away. Permanently.

This is one big regret I have. Not knowing how to deal with my emotions. Hiding behind anger instead of letting myself be vulnerable. The consequences of this 'anger' and 'lashing out' are things I have had to deal with in my recovery, and to this day, and not to sound dramatic, but *forever.*

Let me explain. I lashed out at my friends. My closest

friends that went out of their way to take turns visiting me in the hospital, to take turns spending time with me on the weekends, to take turns keeping me company. And what did I give them in return? A grumpy, complaining, negative attitude. I don't blame them for leaving me.

I lashed out at strangers on the street. Yes, *strangers on the street.* I was that crazy person you'd see walking along the street swearing at myself, and also at anybody that walked by. Yes, I am ashamed to say that I was *that* person. I was holding a lot of vent up anger, frustration and just *anger* at the world, at somebody, at something at whatever caused me to have brain cancer and ruin what was an amazing life.

I knew that *anger* was not doing me any good. It was bad for my health, it was bad for my relationships with my friends and family, it was bad for my recovery!

I tried a lot of things to help me to come to terms with what had happened to me, to accept, to let go of the anger, to be able to *move on* and live life. You see, I knew all of these things, I knew that the anger was bad for me, but I couldn't just *let it go.* So, what I did was I started consulting outside resources; books, articles, and the one thing that really was a turning point for me; Anthony Robbins.

In 2019, I decided to attend the Anthony Robbins Unleash The Power Within seminar in Sydney. It was scary, it was a big move, but I did it. I knew I needed to do something to help myself, and Anthony Robbins seemed like a good idea.

It was a bit daunting to attend such a large event by myself, but I did it. I went in with an open attitude to learning, exploring and meeting new people.

Those 4 days went by so quickly and I utterly enjoyed every single moment. I'm glad I went in alone and scared because that forced me to talk to new people, hear new stories, share my story as well. Also, Anthony Robbins is such an impactful speaker, I really enjoyed hearing him speak about everything from his own journey, to wellness and business. I left the Anthony Robbins seminar with a new take on life, a shift in mindset, an openness to life. It felt so liberating and that feeling stayed with me for the year to come.

Chapter 7: The "bright" side

How do I even start to find the "bright" side in having had brain cancer?

Well, there was one! (There's always a "bright" side if you look hard enough!)

Well, the "bright" side of my brain cancer was that I had my chemotherapy sessions in winter. In winter, it's cold, meaning wearing beanies is normal. So that meant, after receiving chemotherapy and having my hair starting to fall out, I could go beanie shopping because it was beanie season! (that's called looking at the bright side of things).

Boy, did I go beanie shopping! I bought not just one, or two, but three beanies. That way I could wake up and choose which beanie to wear depending on how I was feeling that morning.

To this day, I still own those beanies. They bring back happy memories. Happy memories of my strength in being able to pull through and become the person I am today.

Always see the bright side of things; there's no other side to see!

Chapter 8: Treatments over! Yay! Or nay?

When my treatment was finally over, I felt so happy, I felt that I could start my life again, I could go back to *normal life.*

Boy, was I wrong.

I tried to fit back into "life", but life had moved on, I was "out" for 2 years.

My friends had moved on. Even just walking around the streets, I felt that the TOWN had moved on. There were so many new restaurants, buildings, walkways…

I tried to make new friends by attending lots of meet-ups.

I tried dating through all the dating apps around.

I tried to get back into working.

At one point, I felt like it was easier being in hospital. I had a reason to be doing nothing. I didn't have to think or do anything. My every need was being attended to.

But now, in the real world, I had to figure out what to do with my life; work, friends, free time, health and fitness……..

It was all too much. I was not having a good time.

The two biggest things I wanted, that I felt would solve all of my problems, not necessarily in this order:

1. Find a job, to be financially independent
2. Find a partner, to be loved.

However, I felt that in order to achieve either of these, I needed to first improve my memory.

Chapter 9: On a mission, to improve my memory

Improving my memory was the most important thing on my list during treatment, post treatment, and now, in the current day. I cannot stress enough how important having a working memory is to being able to live a happy and fulfilling life.

I tried many alternative techniques and treatments to improve my memory:

1. *Bowen therapy*; Bowen is a holistic remedial body technique that works on the mechanoreceptors and soft connective tissue (fascia) of the body. Bowen therapy can be used to treat neurological problems. It is gentle and relaxing and does not use forceful manipulation. Bowen therapy is performed on the superficial and deep fascia. The fascia, or soft tissue, is the part of the connective tissue that envelops, separates and influences every organ and tissue in the body. The gentle moves are performed in precise locations to gain maximal influence of the receptors of the nervous system with minimal inputs.

I was recommended to try Bowen therapy. I tried it for about 3 months, going to a session roughly once a week. Aside from it being very relaxing, and spending money that I didn't have, it really didn't have any effects on my memory.

2. *Feldenkrais*; The Feldenkrais Method is a form of somatic education that uses gentle movement and directed attention to improve movement and enhance human functioning. The Feldenkrais Method claims to be successful in training the nervous system to find new pathways around areas of damage, in my case, the damage to my brain.

Upon recommendation from a specialist, I tried a few sessions of Feldenkrais. Unfortunately, I did not feel any benefit from the practice, and did not feel it was for me.

3. *Acupuncture, specifically neuro/scalp acupuncture.* This technique involves the needling of specific areas of the scalp, which help the stimulation of the underlying brain cells.

Again, upon recommendation, I decided to try scalp acupuncture. A few months later, and a few hundred dollars lighter, I felt no difference in my memory function.

4. *Chinese medicine.* Being of Asian background, of course my parents would recommend (inforce) Chinese medicine as a healing avenue. Having tried so many other alternative medicine treatments, and ready to get back to my life, I gave in. I said ok, I'll try Chinese medicine, see if it can heal my broken brain. I gave it a good try. Every morning for roughly 6 months, I drank a bowl of horrible, foul tasting Chinese medicine. To be honest, all it did was make me have very stinky farts. I felt no improvement to my memory.

5. *Supplements;* I was recommended a couple of supplements that would help with my memory issues. I ran it past my treating Doctors, and they were ok with it. So, I started taking USANA CopaPrime+ and Ginkgo Biloba.

USANA CopaPrime+ was marketed as a supplement that would *"Help your mind focus, learn, and make and recall memories with a boost of brain nutrition"* Well, that sounded extremely appealing to me, and exactly what I needed.

Ginkgo biloba extract was marketed as a supplement to help with a range of problems, including anxiety, glaucoma, memory enhancement, dementia, and

Alzheimer's. Of course, memory enhancement stood out for me.

I love to take notes and track my progress. It helps give me a sense of progress. So, when I started taking these supplements, I started a spreadsheet. A very simple spreadsheet with 2 columns for each supplement; Date, Feelings/ Memory moments to note.

The results were varied.

There were moments where I had "memory wins", where I felt that I remembered something that I felt I normally would not.

But then there were also 'memory fail' moments where I would forget something important.

It was a mixed bag, I wasn't convinced that either of these supplements were the magic pill I was looking for to cure my memory problems.

So, in summary, did any of these techniques or treatments work? Did they cure my memory problem? No, none of them "cured" my memory problem. But I do believe they helped in some way. I believe they helped my body, and my healing process along in some way. And it also gave my peace of mind, peace of mind that I had tried *everything*. I was open, I was willing, I was co-operative. Anything and everything that my friends, family, doctors threw at me, I tried. I tried everything so that I would have no regrets of… what if *that* had worked and I didn't try it? No, none of that.

Now, a technique that I have been using since my diagnosis in 2015 to improve my memory, a technique that is incredibly simple and free; daily journaling. On my laptop, I have a file for every single day from my diagnosis in 2015, through to the current day. Yes, *every single day*. Practically, how this worked was, every day, I would have a small notepad with me. In this notepad, I noted things down as they occur throughout the day, anything interesting that happened, or even standard things like what I ate for lunch. Then, at the end of each day, I would transcribe these notes onto a word file on my laptop. Then, in addition to the transcribed notes, I would add anything else I remembered about the day, or how I felt about the day. Just anything really. It was free flow writing, just for me, for my eyes only, so I was free to write whatever I wanted. It was like having a best friend who I could off-load to every night. It was great, and it was exactly what I needed.

Chapter 10: Sharing my story

On 7 December, 2020, I did something that even to this day, I'm not sure how I found the courage to do. I posted my first video on LinkedIn, describing my journey with brain cancer.

From there, I went on to create another 279 videos, ending on 27 October, 2021. I titled this video series "Remembering and Sharing".

My daily journaling notes were simply a recount of my day. Remembering and Sharing, on the other hand, was a collection of video recordings of me narrating instances, learnings and memories of my cancer journey that I felt important to share. Important in the sense that it may help somebody else currently going through brain cancer, or a caregiver of someone going through brain cancer. The video series Remembering and Sharing contained true recounts of my days, living with a brain tumour. Day to day life, from family interactions, tackling work, searching for love… the videos covered it all.

My goal in creating the Remembering and Sharing videos was to spread awareness, and hopefully some compassion of this horrible illness.

I really enjoyed recording these videos everyday. I didn't have any close friends, or close family members with whom I could confide in, so these videos were a form of outlet for me as well, sharing my thoughts and feelings throughout this very scary moment of my life.

In addition to sharing my cancer journey, these videos had an unintended and unexpected outcome. First of all, in creating these videos and speaking into the camera everyday, it increased my self confidence. It increased my public speaking skills. Both of which are *life skills*. I feel grateful, to myself, to have created these videos, and to have invested in my own personal development.

Another unintended and unexpected outcome of my daily videos was reconnecting with friends. My videos were publicly available on my LinkedIn account. After a few weeks of daily videos, I received messages from long lost friends and colleagues, saying hi, or in some cases even sharing that they themselves, or someone close to them had gone through something similar.

It just goes to show, it's not until you share and open up do you realise that you're not alone. There are other people out there suffering as well. Be the leader, be the first to open up, and you'll see, the people you are seeking, they will come.

That was my experience, and I'm so glad I started my video series. I'm so thankful for the reconnections that were made through sharing my story, and for the new connections I made through members of the community who came forward to share their similar stories.

It's a timeless phrase, and it's so true; sharing is caring. It truly is.

I kept a track of the views per post. It was interesting for me to see how many people were viewing my (very amateur) video posts about my life and my experience with cancer.

Chapter 11: Approached by the media

I was approached by a few media sources, to share my story with the public. I note that I did not actively approach the media to share my story. I believe it was an indirect and unintended consequence of my Remembering and Sharing video talks.

I am happy and proud to share my story in the hope that something, anything, even *one* thing I say can help even just that *one* person that is struggling, because, I have been there. I know the loneliness, the pain, the feeling of hopelessness.

The Daily Mail; May 2021

In early 2021, I was approached by The Daily Mail, to share my cancer journey on their platform. The Daily Mail is the highest paid circulation newspaper in the UK.

I was dumbfounded, to say the least, that The Daily Mail wanted to publish a story on me.

From March through to early May I liaised with the editor in charge, sharing my story over the phone and providing images to support the story. The end result is something I am very happy with, and I can honestly say fully captures my cancer journey.

See Appendix 1 for the full story.

That's Life Magazine; Sept 16, 2021, Issue 13

In this article, I talk candidly about my brain cancer journey. I share how despite being unable to return to my "pre-cancer" fast-paced corporate job, that being able to spend my time volunteering helped me along in my recovery, by giving me a sense of purpose in life.

This was printed in a physical magazine. I bought one for myself, as a keep-sake. I'm not sure if any physical copies are still in circulation, however, I have included an image of the article.

See Appendix 2 for an image of the published article.

ZenOnco.io, a cancer care organisation based in India, May 2022

In this article, I share my journey from the beginning; the challenges, the lessons I learnt along the way as well as my sources of motivation and joy, to keep going, to keep fighting. The article ends with what life is like after cancer, and a message to other cancer patients as well as caregivers, to seek out help, to be patient, to show love for oneself, and to each other.

See Appendix 3 for the published article.

Chapter 12: A purpose in life

What is life without a purpose? For me, there is no life without purpose. And coming out of cancer treatment after 2 years, I felt no purpose in my life.

Purpose in life can be defined in different ways by different people, depending on what you value.

For me, a purposeful life include doing work that I find fulfilling, and having a partner to share life's ups and downs with.

Finding work, prior to brain cancer, was something that came very easily for me. I had a good CV, I was personable and knew how to perform well in an interview.

Finding a partner also came easily to me, pre cancer. I knew how to dress to impress and I could hold an intelligent conversation with my date.

Fast forward to present day, i.e post cancer, and the story is very different.

Finding work is very difficult, to say the least, given the 2-year break in my resume whilst I was doing treatment for my brain cancer.

Similarly, finding a partner also became very difficult. It was difficult for me to uphold a conversation with a new date, there was too much new information coming through (name, suburb they live in, place they work at, their hobbies, favourite food, favourite holiday destination, etc. etc.).

Chapter 13a: Finding work

Finding work was something very important to me. Prior to my diagnosis, I was a very high performing individual with a lot of potential to climb the corporate ladder. I knew that with a 2 year break in my CV and with my sub-par memory that I wouldn't be able to go back to the same kind of high-performance roles I used to work in.

I was happy and willing to "take a step back" in terms of seniority and pay in order to get back into the workforce.

In 2015, I very happily accepted a role at Home 789, a specialized real estate company, as a receptionist. This was my first job out of treatment and I was so excited. After my first day, I, sadly, realised that my memory was still causing me difficulties. I share a 'memory fail' as I like to call it relating to this company in the Memory Fail's section.

Employment history from 2015 to 2023:

Company	Position	Tenure
Home789	Executive Assistant	1 month
Global Capital Commercial	Executive Assistant	1 day
ANZ Private	Executive Assistant	1 month
Wealth Creation Advisers	Client Services and Admin Assistant	1 week
Jennings Partners	Executive Assistant	1 week
White and Partners	Team Assistant	1 month
Wise Tech Global	Team Assistant	1 day
UBS	Business Administrator	1 month
Spitfire Paintball & Go Karting	Receptionist and Customer Service	4 months
Flash Painting Services	Customer Service, Appointment Setter	1 day
Save the Children Op Shop	Sales Assistant	3 months
Noni B	Sales Assistant	3 months
Britannica Digital Learning	Sales Consultant	8 months
SuperCare	Customer Service Consultant	1 day

As per my employment history above, that's a count of fourteen jobs over a period of nine years, the shortest tenure being one day and the longest being eight months. It's not something to be proud of. Of the fourteen jobs, there were only three workplaces that I left voluntarily. That leaves eleven of which that I was fired from. If you've ever been fired, you would understand the emotional impact it has on you. Imagine being fired *eleven* times!

Also, take a look at the tenure column. Imagine being employed for one day, *just one day*, and the employer has already figured out there is something wrong with you and they don't want to see you again. That happened to me four times, *four times!*

After every failed attempt at work, I felt absolutely demoralised. It would take me weeks to get back up on my feet and try again. I like to use the analogy of a break-up to describe how this felt.

Chapter 13b: Finding love

I felt like what I needed was to feel loved and needed by someone. I wanted a partner. I wanted a life-long partner. I wanted a loving husband. I made it my mission to find *the one.*

It was tough. Dating is a tough game. My short term memory issues made it even tougher. Meeting new people and holding a conversation, without repeating myself or asking something that was already answered, was so incredibly difficult for me.

I began with the most popular and obvious avenue; dating apps.

Upon searching 'dating apps' in my phone, I realised there were *lots* of dating apps out there, *lots* like about 40. In my time of desperation, I installed and signed up for all of them. *All of them.* I quickly realised why Tinder, Bumble and Coffee Meets Bagel were the tops ones. These ones allowed you to filter your search by age, location, height... factors that are important when looking for *the one.* So, in the end, that's what I was left with, the mainstream dating apps. How many chats, how many dates did I go on? Well, I can tell you! Because of my horrible memory, I actually kept a log of every date I went on, recording the dates name, and things we spoke about. Reason for this is because if the date happened to ask me out for a second date, and if was keen, then I could revert to my notes in order to remember who this date was and what we spoke about, what we did or ate or where we went for a first meet up. Opening up my folder now, named "Dating, No", I went on 59 "no" dates, meaning my current husband was number 60!

As well as the most popular avenue; dating apps, I also tried a couple of other less traditional routes. I wanted to make sure all bases were covered and that I had the best chance of finding *the one* as soon as possible, so I tried speed dating and, also a paid dating service.

The speed dating event I attended left me wondering *who* would ever find their perfect someone at a speed dating event.

In case you've never been to a speed dating even, I will describe how it works. This one I went to was held in a bar, upstairs, the organization must have booked out the section for a couple of hours.

You pay a fee to be part of the event, the one I went to was around $50, from memory. You also get free drinks for the time you're there. The ladies are instructed to sit at a table, and it's the men that move around. You get approx. 5 minutes with each person where can you chat about whatever you like in order to get to know each other a little bit. At the end of each 'session', you write down the person's name if you liked them.

At the end of all the sessions, everyone hands in their piece of paper with the names of the people they liked.

The organisers of the event cross-match the names of those pieces of paper. If there is a match, i.e. if you wrote down someone's name and that person also wrote down your name, then you will be advised and given each other's details to continue conversations.

Now, first of all, how could you determine whether you like someone off the back of a 5 minute conversation? Also, you are forced to chat to *everyone*.

In my desperation to find a partner, I also joined a *dating service*. I don't even remember how I came across it, I think on a flyer or advertisement on the street. Anyway, in my time of desperation, I paid the membership fee, from memory it was around $200. By being a member, you get paired up with someone who fits your description of a perfect partner. And, if after meeting, you are not happy with the date, you are allowed 2 more matches. I thought that sounded like a good deal. So I signed up.

After my first match, I realised my mistake. I was so stupid. Only *after* the fact could I think clearly. Who in this world would pay for a dating service? Would I actually find a handsome, smart, educated man through such a service? NO! The only people who would *pay* for a dating service were, sadly to say, people like *me* at the time. People who could not find anyone. For me, it was because of my disability. For other people, like the first guy I was matched with, is because they are socially awkward.

It was in my desperation to find *the one* that I fell for this.

Chapter 14: Social media

Throughout my treatment and the years following I had (have) a love/ hate relationship with social media.

On the love side, it allowed me to meet and interact with other people who had experienced brain cancer, to understand their journey, their ups and downs, and to feel that I was not alone.

On the hate side, well, seeing posts of my peers out, drinking, having fun, that was hard, because I wasn't there with them. I was (used to be) quite the party gal. Seeing those posts, photos and comments reminded me that that part of my life was over.

Also, seeing posts of my peers being promoted to very senior positions, although being happy for their success was one feeling, sadly, the dominant feeling was one of failure on my behalf, failure to reach anywhere near where my peers were, and the knowledge that because of my brain damage, I will *never* get there.

Social media. It's a two-edged sword.

Chapter 15: Memory fail's

I'd like to conclude my novella with some real life examples of my Memory Fails, as I like to call them, and hence the name of this book. I can now share and talk about these, and perhaps laugh at some of them, which I am grateful for, grateful to have some out of all of this a better and stronger person. However, having said that, these are absolutely true accounts of the day-to-day issues I had to deal with, and am still dealing with (but to a lesser extent). The 'Memory Fail' in me is permanent, but I've learnt how to cope with it in a positive light.

Memory fail; 1

It's 2015, I'm in the hospital for one of my chemotherapy rounds. As I was packing for my 3-night stay at the hospital, my mother suggested that I leave my phone at home. Leaving my phone at home is not something I would normally do, so I forgot that that is what I did.

I arrived at the hospital and settled into my room. I was taken to do some scans, and after coming back from those scans, I couldn't find my phone and I remembered seeing a nurse leave my room as I was coming back in. I immediately assumed that the nurse had stolen my phone. I called a nurse over to say that my phone was stolen and I suspected it was the nurse that had just left the room.

The alarm was sounded. At that point, I borrowed a nurse's phone to call my mother to tell her my phone had been stolen. My mother answered, 'no, you left your phone at home'. It was at that point that I remembered my mother had forced me to leave it at home in case someone steals it.

My memory found it hard to remember a non-routine action. This is something I still struggle with today. And, needless to say, I was very embarrassed to call the nurse over *again*, to tell her no one had stole my phone, I had left my phone at home.

Memory fail; 2

I'm on the train. I could not remember where I was going, or who I was seeing. How did I solve it, or try to solve it? I looked in my handbag for clues, I looked in my notepad for clues, I looked in my phone for clues, searching for text messages and emails. Surely something in there would give me a clue as to where I was going and who I was planning on seeing. Surely!

This technique, 'looking for clues' is something I still use today. Due to my damaged memory, it has become a habit for me to write things done, even things that may seem non-important. I write everything down in my notepad when I'm out, and on my laptop on a word file when I'm home. Then, at the end of each day, I transfer all of my notes in my notepad onto my word file on my laptop.

I have a word document for every single day from my diagnosis through to today. These files help me. They have helped me immensely in the past, where I am trying to remember where I went, who I saw, what I ate… I look through my daily word files to figure out where I have been, where I have gone, who I have seen.

I call it doing detective work on my own life. It sounds extreme to have a word file for every day since 2015, but it's a coping mechanism, it's an external memory drive for me, to compensate for my broken, internal memory.

Memory fail; 3

There was one day (no, probably not just *one* day) where I couldn't remember whether I had had dinner yet. Yes, a very odd problem to have.

What did I do?

I consulted my stomach, do I feel full?

I went to the kitchen to see if the dishes had been done recently, or were there dirty dishes in the sink?

I looked in the rubbish bin; were there any recent food scraps in there to indicate I had done some food preparation?

At that point, I knew my memory was and would potentially be 'broken' for the rest of my life. But I felt a slight, very slight feeling of proudness that I could think of ways to 'detective-work' a solution to my problem.

Memory fail; 4

I'm on a date and, all of a sudden I couldn't remember which suburb I was in, what we were doing, and what we had done previously in the evening. I voiced it, 'where are we again?' and (understandably) my date gave me an incredibly weird look. I thought, oh no, another one that's going to ghost me.

But no, I was happily surprised, he stuck around, and by the way, this is my now husband.

Memory fail; 5

I had just started a new job (my first job post treatment actually). The role was as per my previous background, so I thought I would be fine, or even more than fine. I was very wrong, I made many mistakes, and was told off many times.

The biggest mistake I made, which, upon thinking about it really demonstrates the extent of my brain damage. I was the executive assistant at a company. I was instructed to order a new boardroom table, which I did. The following week, a boardroom table arrived. However, a couple of days later, *another* boardroom table arrived.

Needless to say, my boss was very confused. I knew it was my fault, I had accidently ordered *two* boardroom tables because I had forgotten I had already ordered the first one. Instead of owning up to it, I did a naughty, I just played dumb and said that the delivery company obviously got it wrong. Not my finest moment.

Memory fail; 6

I made chicken drumsticks for dinner. I only used half the pack because I remember my husband said to leave him half, he wanted to make something with it.

We were eating dinner and my husband asked if there was more chicken. I said no, I only cooked half the pack because I saved the other half for him, as per his request. He said no.

Then, upon thinking about it, he said that *last week* about *last weeks chicken*. Last week, I had made chicken soup and he made fried chicken with the left over chicken.

So not only do I forget things, I get my memories jumbled up too.

Memory fail; 7

I love massages. I have a regular place I go to. One day, I was standing outside my favourite massage place looking at the board trying to decide which massage I wanted.

The lady saw me looking at the massage menu and laughingly said 'another one?', which is when I realised/presumed I had already had one that day and laughed (faking it) at her comment and walked away embarrassed.

Needless to say, I felt embarrassed and ashamed of myself for having such a big memory fail. Not only did my brain forget, but my body forgot too. Surely, I would have felt relaxed and that would have sent signals to my brain and memory that I had already had a massage. Those were the thoughts going through my head as I (very ashamedly) walked away from the massage shop.

Memory fail; 8

My brother and his wife had a baby. I went shopping for a baby gift. It was mid-November so I also bought a Christmas present for my brothers other kid, my niece, as well.

I delivered everything together and told him that too, that I was pre-gifting a Christmas gift for his daughter because we might not see each other again before Christmas.

THEN, just a few days later, I put on my to-do list to look for a Christmas present for my niece and new-born nephew. I bought two lovely plush toys for my niece and nephew, then called my brother to arrange a Christmas catch up so I can give his children their presents.

He said I had already given presents. I was confused. Then the NEXT day, out of nowhere, I remembered, he was correct, I had indeed already bought presents.

Chapter 16: Gratefulness

I am grateful for the challenges I have faced. Despite the pain, I am grateful for how the challenges I have faced have made me into the person I am today. I can say wholeheartedly that going through cancer is life changing, in a positive way. It allows you to appreciate life, I mean, *really* appreciate life. It allows you to appreciate the small things and not fret the big things. It's helped me to learn to live in the moment. Don't wait for tomorrow, do it now. Don't save every cent, splurge on yourself every now and then, you deserve it. Live in the now. Love yourself. Love your friends and family. Be a kind person and be a giving person to society. Life is short, look forwards, move forwards, and remember to smile.

Closing note

The 'memory fails' I have shared range from my diagnosis back in 2014, all the way through to current day, 2024.

I am a work in progress. And, I have progressed. I truly have. From cancer diagnosis in 2014 to current day, 2024, I've trained my memory from not being able to remember whether I'd eaten breakfast, to being able to write this book! I went from lonely and depressed, to now happily married.

My message to you is, please, have faith in yourself, surround yourself with those that truly, deeply, unconditionally care for you… that's all you need to fulfill your dreams.

Dedication and Thank you's

I dedicate this book to anyone that has been diagnosed with a brain tumour, or has experienced brain trauma, as well as their friends, family and loved ones.

A sincere thank you to the Doctors at Royal North Shore Hospital (Dr Back, Dr Bligh, Dr Wheeler), the Synapse team, and last but not least, my family, friends and forever loving husband, Sam.

Appendix 1. The Daily Mail, May 2021

How young woman who was living her dream life lost her high-flying 100k-a-year job AND her long-term boyfriend after shock diagnosis at age 26

- Linda Lee had it all: a high-flying career, long-term partner and a six-figure salary
- But her world was shattered by a shock brain cancer diagnosis at the age of 26
- The impact of her tumour left the Sydney businesswoman with memory loss
- Treatment was successful but she lost everything and is unable to return to work
- Ms Lee has revealed how a self-help guru helped her through her darkest days

A high-flying businesswoman has revealed how a shock brain cancer diagnosis saw her lose her six-figure salary, long-term partner and future career.

At 26, Linda Lee was excelling in every aspect of life, earning $100,000 a year from her job in financial services while planning to relocate to **London** with her boyfriend of three years.

But her world came crashing down when doctors discovered a tumour the size of a golf ball in her brain.

Treatment proved successful, but damage caused by the tumour left the Sydney saleswoman with acute memory loss which has made it impossible for her to return to work.

Now 33, Ms Lee told Daily Mail Australia how advice from a self-help guru saw her through her darkest days - and how volunteering with refugees has given her newfound purpose in life.

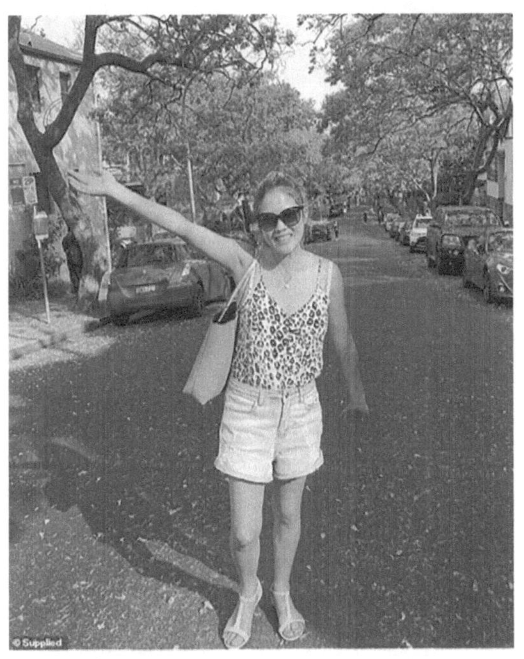

Image of Linda Lee, 'living the life'

At 26, Sydney businesswoman Linda Lee (pictured) had it all - a high-flying career, a long-term partner and a six-figure salary

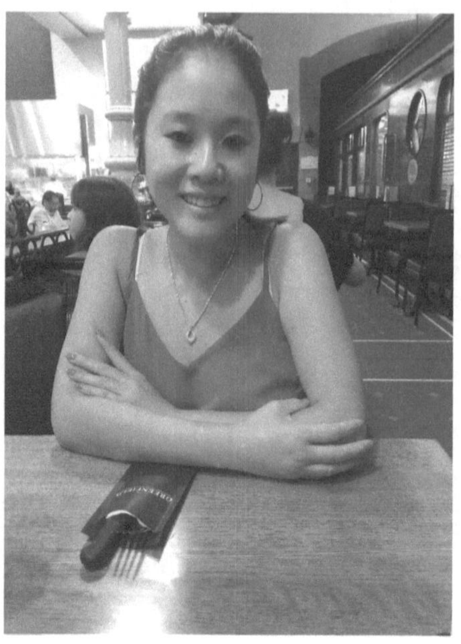

Image of Linda Lee pre diagnosis

Ms Lee's world came crashing down when doctors discovered a tumour the size of a golf ball lodged in the prefontal cortex of her brain

Before her diagnosis in the winter of 2015, Ms Lee began to suffer from memory loss which left her unable to remember instructions for simple tasks and confused about conversations she'd had moments earlier.

She also experienced hallucinations which made her believe she was speaking to someone who was not really there.

Ms Lee went to see a GP, who referred her for scans

and a biopsy which showed a germinoma was growing in her prefrontal cortex.

A germinoma is a rare form of cancer that originates in sex cells that failed to leave the brain when it forms in the womb.

'It was devastating,' Ms Lee said of her diagnosis.

Doctors prescribed an 18 month course of chemotherapy and radiation which eliminated all traces of cancer.

But the impact of the tumour changed Ms Lee's life forever.

Image 4

Treatment proved successful, but damage caused by the tumour left Ms Lee (pictured after her biopsy) with acute memory loss which has made it impossible for her to return to work

What is a germinoma?

A germinoma is a rare form of cancer that is most often found in the brain of children between the ages of 10 and 19 years.

The cancer originates in germ cells, which are actually sex cells that fail to leave the brain when the foetus is still in utero.

There are two main types - germinomas and

non-germinomatous germ cell tumors - which respond differently to treatment.

Symptoms depend on where the tumor develops in the brain and its size.

Common telltale signs include caused by a swelling of the brain include fatigue, vomiting, headache, behavioural changes, and difficulty with movements or vision.

Source: Children's Cancer Australia

The severe memory loss doctors say she will live with for the rest of her life forced her to abandon her career and left her unable to hold down another job.

'I went from earning $100,000 a year to being fired from countless jobs one after another. It was really difficult for me to accept that that part of my life is gone,' Ms Lee said.

When her partner discovered she would be unable to move to the UK, he ended their relationship.

Ms Lee said she developed depression and experienced suicidal thoughts after her condition forced her to move back to her family home and push friends and loved ones away.

'Even now it's hard for me to see my peers and where they're at,' she said.

'I think about where I could be if this hadn't happened to me.'

[image 10]

Ms Lee said she developed depression and experienced suicidal thoughts after her condition forced her to move back to her family home and push friends and loved ones away

She finally found peace after attending a seminar hosted by American life coach Tony Robbins, whose advice helped her to 'stop seeing herself as a victim'.

In late 2020 she started volunteering with Save the Children and Core Community Services, a support group that helps refugees find jobs in Australia.

Despite being unpaid, Ms Lee said the work has given her newfound fulfilment.

'I love being busy and it makes me feel worthy. It's given me a sense of purpose,' she said.

Ms Lee has shared her story to encourage Australians to support Australia's Biggest Morning Tea, a fundraising event run by the NSW Cancer Council which takes place on May 27.

For more information on germinomas of the brain and central nervous system, please visit the Australian Cancer Council or Children's Cancer Australia.

Appendix 2. That's Life Magazine; Sept 16, 2021, Issue 13

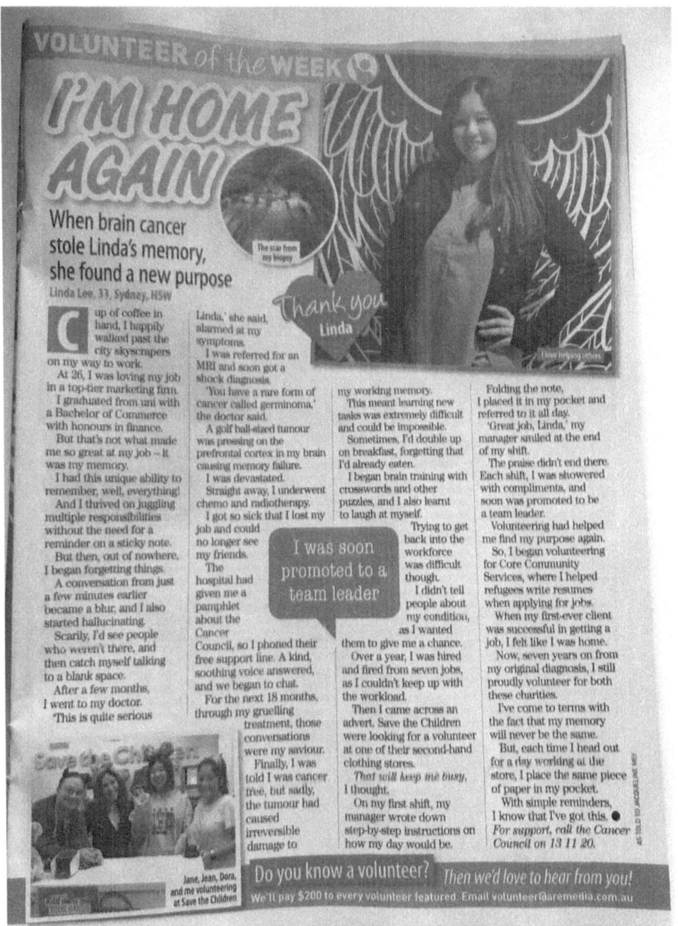

Cup of coffee in hand, I happily walked past the city skyscrapers on my way to work.

At 26, I was loving my job in a top-tier marketing firm.

I graduated from uni with a Bachelor of Commerce with honours in finance.

But that's not what made me so great at my job – it was my memory.

I had this unique ability to remember, well, everything!

And I thrived on juggling multiple responsibilities without the need for a reminder on a sticky note.

But then, out of nowhere, I began forgetting things.

A conversation from just a few minutes earlier became a blur, and I also started hallucinating.

Scarily, I'd see people who weren't there, and then catch myself talking to a blank space.

After a few months, I went to my doctor.

'This is quite serious Linda,' she said, alarmed at my symptoms.

I was referred for an MRI and soon got a shock diagnosis.

'You have a rare form of cancer called germinoma,' the doctor said.

A golf ball-sized tumour was pressing on the prefrontal cortex in my brain causing memory failure.

I was devastated.

Straight away, I underwent chemo and radiotherapy.

I got so sick that I lost my job and could no longer see my friends.

The hospital had given me a pamphlet about the Cancer Council, so I phoned their free support line. A kind, soothing voice answered, and we began to chat.

For the next 18 months, through my gruelling treatment, those conversations were my saviour.

Finally, I was told I was cancer free, but sadly, the tumour had caused irreversible damage to my working memory.

This meant learning new tasks was extremely difficult and could be impossible.

Sometimes, I'd double up on breakfast, forgetting that I'd already eaten.

I began brain training with crosswords and other puzzles, and I also learnt to laugh at myself.

Trying to get back into the workforce was difficult though.

I didn't tell people about my condition, as I wanted them to give me a chance.

Over a year, I was hired and fired from seven jobs, as I couldn't keep up with the workload.

Then I came across an advert. Save the Children were looking for a volunteer at one of their second-hand clothing stores.

That will keep me busy, I thought.

On my first shift, my manager wrote down step-by-step instructions on how my day would be.

Folding the note, I placed it in my pocket and referred to it all day.

'Great job, Linda,' my manager smiled at the end of my shift.

The praise didn't end there. Each shift, I was showered with compliments, and soon was promoted to be a team leader.

Volunteering had helped me find my purpose again.

So, I began volunteering for Core Community Services, where I helped refugees write resumes when applying for jobs.

When my first-ever client was successful in getting a job, I felt like I was home.

Now, seven years on from my original diagnosis, I still proudly volunteer for both these charities.

I've come to terms with the fact that my memory will never be the same.

But, each time I head out for a day working at the store, I place the same piece of paper in my pocket.

With simple reminders, I know that I've got this. ●

For support, call the Cancer Council on 13 11 20.

That's Life magazine

Appendix 3. ZenOnco.io, May 2022

https://zenonco.io/cancer/linda-lee-brain-cancer-survivor/

Linda Lee (Brain Cancer Survivor)

May 30, 2022

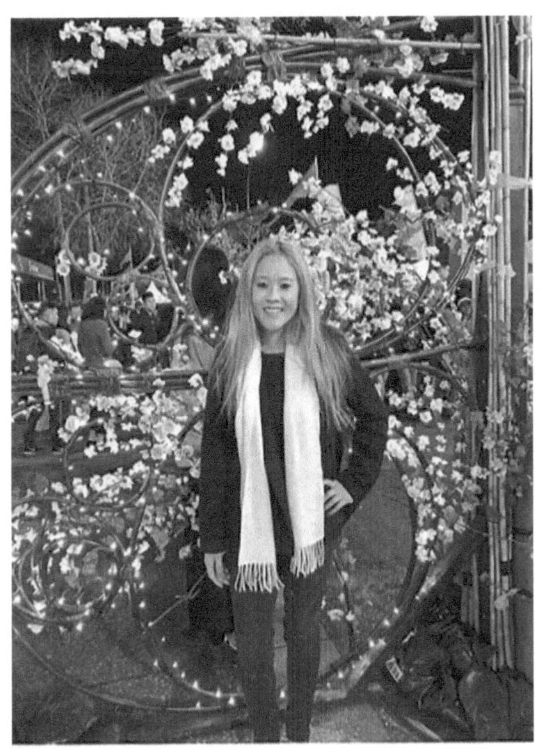

The very first sign

The very first symptom that something is wrong was my memory. I used to have an amazing memory. And then all of a sudden, I just started forgetting things. I couldn't do my work properly. I was working in the client services and financial services market research company, which involves a lot of memory work, and a lot of multitasking, and I was doing well at my job. And then all of a sudden, I started forgetting to do things, and my manager got really angry at me.

I even had hallucinations. For instance, I'd be walking along the street by myself thinking I'm talking to someone, and when I turned around to find the streets empty. So I went to my GP and I told her my symptoms. She straightaway sent me to get an MRI. When the MRI came back showing a tumour in my brain which was sized as big as a golf ball. The part of the brain affected was the hypothalamus. Tumour was growing on the part of the brain responsible for working memory. And that's why I was experiencing memory issues.

But the doctor told me the good news that the German reacts very well to treatment. So it's highly treatable. So I started my treatment, which was chemotherapy and radiation therapy. I did three rounds of chemotherapy and a month of radiation therapy. And thankfully, the treatment was successful.

Side effects and challenges

I've been cancer-free since 2017. However, I feel that my cancer journey really started after my treatment, because then it was about trying to get back fit back into life. Although I was cancer-free and no longer had a tumour in my brain, it had done permanent damage to my working memory. So even now, my memory is not perfect, and I'm not able to work. I'm not able to do the same kind of work I used to do.

I tried to get back into the workforce. And I tried roles that were a few levels down easier than what I used to do. And I still couldn't handle it. I went through eight jobs in the space of 18 months. The shortest tenure was a couple of hours. And the longest tenure was three months. And the reason why I kept getting fired from all of these roles, is my memory. So after going through all of that for two years, trying and then getting fired. I finally decided that this just wasn't working. So I tried something different. I saw an ad for volunteering. So I started volunteering, and it worked out. I'm very happy about that.

Support group/caregiver

My support system was definitely my family. My mother, my father, and my older brother. They were in and out of the hospital visiting me and helping me. I wouldn't have been able to do it without them. I was at the Royal North Shore Hospital in Sydney. And I feel that the SIRT, the neurosurgeon, and the oncology doctors, were all very good, very knowledgeable, and I felt like I was in good hands.

Source of motivation and joy

Things that made me happy and healthy, are definitely having family there. Just such as having them, not just for getting help but just for having their presence. So when I was in the hospital during my treatment, when you wake up until you go to sleep, it's a really long day if you don't have any visitors. I was lucky enough to always have someone there with me, which was really helpful. Yes, so you know, there are times when you feel that it's too much to bear, but you still don't give up. You keep on working on those days. So what was the thing that motivated you and kept you going on such days?

So on a really bad day, what motivated me to keep going and not give up was just the belief that it was going to be better. Life can't just be like this. It's got to get better. And so that motivated me to keep going forwards.

Lessons that I learned

I think that cancer has positively changed me. My journey went from hating life to valuing life. It has brought me closer to my family and I shouldn't take them for granted. I got some very important life lessons. Number one is to enjoy life because it's short. So don't say for a rainy day, just if you want to do something, or you want to. Just do it. Don't wait, because you don't know what's going to happen between now and then. That's one of the main things. Another lesson is that family is very important. Keep them close and keep them happy. Yeah, that's true. Family is the biggest supporter we find during those times.

Life after cancer

I think I just made a conscious effort to eat more healthily because it couldn't hurt. More healthy eating and a more healthy lifestyle. So healthy eating and exercise are what I adopted. I even started volunteering. So I apparently have two volunteer roles. One helping the children selling secondhand clothes, and another one at

Community Services as a refugee youth mentor. I've been volunteering for about a year or so now.

Message for other cancer patients and caregivers

I want to tell other cancer patients to be strong and to seek out others who are on a similar journey. Because it's just so important to have people to talk to. And it's even better if those people can actually empathise with what you're going through.

And to the caregivers, I would say, just be patient. I know it's hard, but don't judge and don't get frustrated at people for things they can't help because then it just makes it worse. For me, for example, my memory was horrible. So when my caregivers would be like I've already told you that. Caregivers shouldn't be saying things like that, because I used to fall into a period of depression for days. So, I ask the caregivers to be patient.

9 798765 200162